VITAMIN C AND PAIN, JERRY'S HOSPITAL VISIT

Jerry Scherer

DEDICATION

First, I want to dedicate this book to my daughter, Jacquelyn, for her diligence in seeking a cure for her kitties. She would not have stumbled upon molecular medicine, without this effort.

I also dedicate this book to all of the people who spend their lives, usually for minimal pay, trying to help a brainwashed world see the value in nutrition.

And lastly, I would like to salute all the great women and men who have worked so hard to try to educate a brainwashed world and have since passed on to the other side.

CONTENTS

Acknowledgments i

1 Headed to the Hospital 9

2 Surgery 10

3 They Transported Me 12

4 Please Give Me Pain-Killers 14

5 A Few Facts about Vitamin C 15

6 Getting My Stomach Pumped 17

7 I Took 10 Vitamin C Pills 19

8 Someone Died from Pain 21

9 "No Way, I'm Feeling Better" 22

10 Tom Selleck 24

11 Listening to Tunes 26

12 Timed-Release Vitamin C 27

13 The Discovery of Vitamin C 30

14 Famous Vitamin C Doctors 31

Disclaimer 35

About the Author 36

ACKNOWLEDGMENTS

I especially want to thank the Riordan Clinic for making their videos, and other publications available without charge, for without their dedication I would still be sick.

I want to thank Google for making it possible to read publications that have been hidden from the public for years.

Jerry Scherer

Chapter One

Headed to the Hospital

In the summer of 2012, a hernia, which I had had for a number of years, strangulated. If any of you do not know what this means, it basically means pain, fever, and a life-threatening situation. After allowing the fever to get the best of me I decided to go to the hospital. It was about 9:00 in the evening when I arrived and they immediately admitted me. Since I had eaten a few hours before, they put a tube down my throat and pumped my stomach, which felt worse than the hernia.

Chapter Two

Surgery

I went to surgery and got the thing repaired. When I awoke, I was in the recovery room. I'm sure that anyone who has had surgery, surely knows that, when you wake up after surgery, it feels like you've been beaten in the head and are just waking up from this bad beating. The recovery room nurse (God bless all of them.) came over and asked, "How are you doing?" Well, even as sick as I was, I wanted to say "Never better," but, being sick as hell I said, "OK," which was a lie. All of you, if you've had surgery, know what I mean. The nurse asked me if I needed something for pain. (Why do they even ask such a thing?) All I can figure is that they haven't ever had surgery or they must say it

because it is in the "Golden"
rule book for nurses. It's not
in any rule book for doctors,
that's for sure. When the nurse
asked me if I wanted some pain
medicine I said "Yes" so timidly
that she had to ask again. The
reason for everyone saying yes so
timidly is because they know how
bad drugs are and they don't want
the nurse to think that they are
drug addicts, but drug addicts
are the only ones that say it so
timidly, so they know that you
are a drug addict anyway. (I'm
just kidding.) So I got the good
drugs. It must have been morphine
because I was immediately walking
on streets of gold. I knew for
sure that I had just walked into
heaven.

Chapter Three

They Transported Me

They transported me to my room. I knew it was a transporter, like the one on Star Trek, because I could hear distorted voices and I could see that I was traveling through the clouds.

As I woke up in my room, I made the mistake of moving. As I did, it felt like I had just fallen on that crossbar on a bicycle. By the way, why in the world do girls have no crossbars but boys do? After I lay still for a few minutes, the pain settled down and I was able to push the button for the nurse. It seemed like the nurse took an hour to get there. When she arrived, she smiled at me as if she was the one that was in pain. I realized that she was trying to empathize but drugs were what I really wanted and the fact that she was trying to show empathy wasn't doing anything for my pain. She said, "I'll be right back."

Meanwhile, a woman, (I'm not sure who she was.) came into my room and asked me questions about my stay. (Why do they do that when you have just gotten out of the butcher shop?) Anyway, she said, "It looks like you will need to stay here, at least another day." I thought, "As long as they put the knives away, I'll stay."

Chapter Four

Please Give Me Pain-Killers

After waiting for two years, or so it seemed, I pushed the buzzer again. The same nurse walked into my room and said, "Oh, I'm so sorry. I got side tracked. I'll be right back." I waited and waited for her to return. It seemed as if were forever. By now, the pain was so bad, tears were trickling down my cheeks. I could hear my nurse, or some nurse, in the hall, giving orders to other nurses. I guess they were very busy that day and didn't have enough help.

I don't know why, to this day, that I grabbed my pants, which were hanging over a chair by my bed, but I did. I reached into my pants pocket and pulled out a handful of pills.

Chapter Five

A Few Facts about Vitamin C

Let me take you back in time for a moment. For some time before this, my daughter had been studying Vitamin C. She told me that Vitamin C was the best antioxidant because it had two electrons that could be donated to neutralize toxins. Since it had two electrons to donate, it was twice as powerful as any other antioxidant. I know all of this sounds silly but we are made of molecules and bad ones get neutralized by good ones. She told me that Vitamin C was a pain killer and I thought, "Well, maybe a little, but nothing beats morphine." She told me lots of things that Vitamin C could do. I'll go into some of these things later, but I want to continue my hospital story first.

When I reached into my pocket and grabbed the handful of Vitamin C pills, there were 10 of them. I finally got my bed in an upright position so I could pull the tray over closer and pour a glass of water.

Chapter Six

Getting My Stomach Pumped

Let me back up again for a minute. I don't know if any of you ever had your stomach pumped before, but putting the tube down your throat is a panic that I could never describe to you with words. However, I'll try. They have you drink some kind of motor oil as they slide this tube down your throat. They keep telling you to drink while you're gagging, to beat all hell, and when you stop, they yell at you and tell you to keep drinking. It was the day after the tube was gone but it felt like it was still in there. My throat was so sore that I couldn't swallow at all. I just laid there and drooled. Here I am, thinking I'm going to take a drink of water. I put the cup up to my mouth to take a very, very, very little sip of water and try to swallow, and down my wind pipe it goes. Right then, the biggest baddest kick boxer in the world came in my room and began kicking me in the gut, or that's what it felt like. I coughed and coughed and coughed. I tried with all of my might not to cough, but I kept coughing and coughing and coughing. My gut burned. I knew I had ripped out all of my stitches or whatever they used to repair my hernia. After what seemed like forever, I stopped coughing. I'm not sure how long it took to figure out how to swallow water without coughing but I finally did and I took the Vitamin C pills.

Chapter Seven

I Took 10 Vitamin C Pills

I can't really tell you why I wanted to take the vitamin C pills. Maybe, deep in my mind, I thought that they would help me. Or, maybe I was just delirious from the pain. But I do remember taking them. It's not like I hadn't ever taken any Vitamin C pills before. In fact, I had taken lots of them; not because I was convinced that they would help me, but because my daughter was taking them. Since I knew she was well-read about a lot of things, I, at least, partially trusted her.

I took ten pills 1000 milligrams (1-gram each) of time-released Vitamin C, I'm not sure how much of the vitamin C dissolves right away it just says that it dissolves in 6 to 8 hours. Now, remember what I said about Vitamin C? It is the greatest antioxidant that there is, so it has twice the power to neutralize toxins as anything else does. When I took all of those pills, here is what was happening; the toxins in my body were being neutralized. At this point, you may be saying, "What does any of this have to do with anything?"

Chapter Eight

Someone Died from Pain

As I lay in the bed, I heard the blue light special thing. (No, wait. That's K Mart.) I heard the Code Blue. (Or is it Red?) Anyway, I heard a lot of commotion in the hall and all of these people, who looked like nurses and doctors were running down the hall. I guess someone else did not get their pain meds either and decided to just die.

Chapter Nine

"No Way, I'm Feeling Better"

As I lay there, I started to feel better. No, better is not the correct word. I started to feel great. Now, I wasn't thinking that Vitamin C is the almighty pain-killer, at this point. I really didn't think about it at all. I just knew that I was feeling great, so I sat up in bed. I looked at the water and had a flashback so I left it alone. Then I sat up on the edge of the bed. I needed to go to the bath room so I stood up and pushed my IV cart into the bathroom. Well, it really wasn't a bathroom since it didn't have a bathtub, but you get where I was. When I finished up, I looked into the mirror. I saw a person who needed the undertaker. I looked at myself and thought, "I need to clean myself up." I washed my face, wet down my hair and combed it. I pushed the IV cart back over to my bed and decided to get dressed.

At this point you must be thinking that I am just crazy but the things that I am telling you are the plain facts. I got dressed, which was a task, in itself, because, to get my shirt on, I had to lift the IV bag off the stand to get it through my shirt sleeve. (You get the picture.)

Chapter Ten

Tom Selleck

As I stood there, thinking I needed to get rid of the IV bag, the nurse walked in with a syringe full of pain-killer. She looked at me and her mouth dropped to the floor, as it were. She just stood there for the longest time, not knowing what to say. Then she walked over to the door and yelled "Hey, come here." Within a couple of moments, there were a number of nurses in the room, looking at me. My nurse said, "Look at him." They all looked, in a mysterious way, as if to be saying, "What?" She said it again. "Will you look at that?" Then, one of the nurses said, "Tom Selleck." I had to say, I was flattered at that remark. I guess she was shocked that I was up and dressed, I simply asked my nurse if she would take the IV out of my arm. She said, "Yes." She went to a cabinet got a few things out of it and then came over and removed it. When I looked up everyone was gone.

I was feeling exceptionally great even though, not even 12 hours before, I had had major surgery and not just major surgery. I had an infection from tissue strangulation. At first, the doctors thought that part of my intestine was pinched through the hole and that was why I had a high fever and my blood pressure was so high. After the surgery, my doctor told me that it was fat that had pushed through my torn muscle and it had gotten caught and infected.

Chapter Eleven

Listening to Tunes

The nurse had just removed my IV. I felt great. I grabbed my phone, plugged in my headset, turned on some tunes and called Cathy, my sweet girl friend, whom I love with all of my heart. I told her that I wanted to come home. She said, "I thought you were going to stay." I said, "No, I'm feeling great." I guess, after the surgery, I had talked with her, but I don't remember it.

As I waited for Cathy to pick me up, I walked up and down the hall. Each time I passed the nurse's station, they looked at me in disbelief. I'm sure they were wondering how in the world I went from deathly sick to feeling so great, in such a short time.

Chapter Twelve

Timed-Release Vitamin C

I took timed-release Vitamin C here is the exact brand that I took.

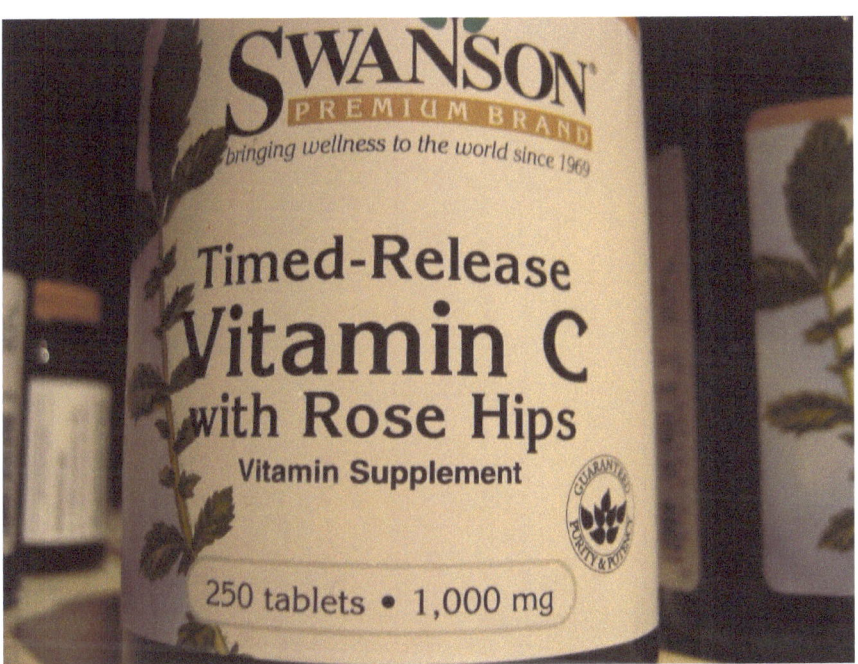

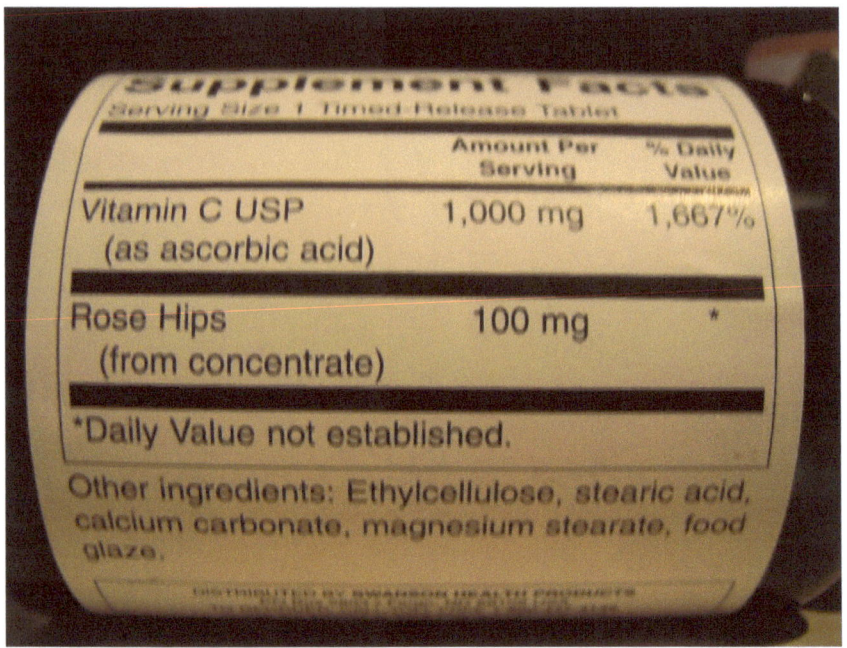

The pill does not dissolve until it is in the small intestine and then it begins to dissolve slowly. It takes hours to be completely dissolved which releases the Vitamin C.

This Vitamin C is a pain-killer when taken orally in high enough doses. It stops the inflammation that is caused from the trauma of the knife blade. It killed the infection that I had from the tissue strangulation and it neutralized the poison flowing through my system from being put to sleep. I don't know if any other Vitamin C would work because I have only ever used this time release Vitamin C from Swanson's.

If I ever get an injury again, that would require surgery, I would like to find a doctor that would let me take vitamin C pills and also use Vitamin C via I-V and do the surgery while I'm awake. I think it would work and I'm willing to try it.

There is a lot of information on the internet that you can read about Vitamin C.

Chapter Thirteen

The Discovery of Vitamin C

Vitamin C was actually discovered by the British in 1753 when they realized that Scurvy was caused by malnutrition, but it wasn't given the name Vitamin C until later. The British navy started giving their sailors lime juice in 1795 to prevent Scurvy.

The Vitamin C molecule was discovered in 1930 by Albert Szent-Györgyi, a Hungarian scientist.

Chapter Fourteen

Famous Vitamin C Doctors

Dr Fredrick Klenner, M.D.

Dr Fredrick Klenner was the first to use high doses of Vitamin C intravenously.

From 1943-1947, he treated and cured 41 cases of Viral Pneumonia with high doses of I-V Vitamin C.

From 1948-1949, he cured every Polio case that was brought to him. (More than 50.)

On June 10,1949, at the annual session of the American Medical Association in Atlantic City, New Jersey, he presented his work on I-V Vitamin C and Polio. When he was done, they just moved on, as if he hadn't even spoken.

Here are some of the things he cured with Vitamin C:

Alcoholism, Arthritis, Atherosclerosis, Chronic Fatigue,

Leukemia, High cholesterol, infections, Corneal ulcer, heavy-metal poisoning, Glaucoma, Diabetes, burns, Rocky Mountain Spotted Fever, Heat stroke, bladder infections, ruptured intervertebral discs, surgery complications, Tetanus, Trichinosis, venomous bites from spiders or snakes and Multiple Sclerosis.

Here is a website that talks about Fredrick Klenner's work, in more detail.

http://www.doctoryourself.com/klennerbio.html

Dr Robert F. Cathcart III M.D.

Dr Cathcart figured out how much Vitamin C could be taken orally to bowel tolerance with each kind of disease.

He also used IV Vitamin C for almost everything imaginable and recorded the results as any research scientist would.

Here is a website that talks about Dr Cathcart's work, in more detail.

http://www.doctoryourself.com/titration.html

Dr Linus Pauling, PhD.

Linus Pauling was a two time Nobel prize winner.

He wrote,

"Vitamin C and the Common Cold"

"Cancer and Vitamin C" (with Ewan Cameron, M.D.)

"How to Live Longer and Feel Better"

Here is a website that talks about Linus Pauling's work, in more detail.

http://lpi.oregonstate.edu/infocenter/vitamins/vitaminC/

DISCLAIMER

I am not a doctor. I am merely telling you a true story about an event that happened in my life. If you are in need of medical advice, seek a medical doctor for help.

ABOUT THE AUTHOR

Jerry Scherer works in the Geothermal Heat Pump industry and is known by the name Geojerry. After getting deathly sick, his daughter, Jacquelyn, discovered what Vitamin C can do. Along with that and other nutrition, it brought him back from the edge of death.
Jerry has 4 children and 4 grandchildren. He lives in Kent, Ohio.

www.ingramcontent.com/pod-product-compliance
Lightning Source LLC
Chambersburg PA
CBHW050904290526
45792CB00002B/694